Stroke Recovery Roadmap

A Holistic Guide to Achieving Optimal Wellness and Fulfillment for Patients and Their Support Network

Brenda Alderson

Table of Contents

INTRODUCTION

Within the expansive realm of healthcare, few diagnoses resonate with as much gravity, uncertainty, and emotional intensity as the term "stroke." As the author of "Stroke Recovery Roadmap," my journey as a vascular neurologist has been interwoven with countless narratives of individuals and families grappling with the aftermath of this life-altering event. It is with a profound sense of responsibility and empathy that I embark on this literary journey, seeking to offer guidance, understanding, and a compass for those navigating the challenging terrain of stroke recovery.

A stroke, at its core, represents a sudden and often catastrophic disruption of blood flow to the brain. This interruption manifests in a multitude of ways, leaving a trail of physical, cognitive, and emotional complexities in its wake. It is a medical emergency, a call to action, for the brain, with its unyielding demand for oxygen and nutrients, is exquisitely susceptible to even the briefest deprivation.

Yet, within this seemingly singular medical event, lies a tapestry of diversity. Strokes do not adhere to a one-size-fits-all model. Instead, they emerge in a kaleidoscope of forms, each shaped by its underlying cause and characterized by its unique repercussions. Ischemic strokes, the result of blood clots obstructing cerebral blood vessels, dance to a different tune than their hemorrhagic counterparts, born from the rupture of vessels within the brain, leading to bleeding. These nuances underscore the intricacy of the recovery journey, as each stroke type necessitates tailored strategies and interventions.

In the aftermath of a stroke, individuals and their families often find themselves thrust into a bewildering, unfamiliar landscape. Hospitalizations, medical procedures, and an overwhelming surge of emotions become the new normal. It is a time when questions seem to multiply, and the path forward appears shrouded in an impenetrable fog of uncertainty.

It is here that the significance of recovery guidance is laid bare. It is not a mere repository of statistics and facts; it is a lifeline—a beacon amidst the darkness. It offers clarity when confusion reigns, it instills hope when despair looms, and it provides a roadmap when the future remains obscure. Recovery guidance underscores a fundamental truth: the voyage to healing is not a solitary one; it is a collective endeavor. With the right guidance, stroke survivors, their families, and caregivers can embark on a path toward rejuvenation and renewal.

This comprehensive guide is meticulously crafted to serve as an unwavering companion on the journey of stroke recovery. Whether you stand as a recent survivor grappling with the profound challenges that have materialized, a family member navigating the intricate terrain of caregiving, or a healthcare professional seeking to deepen your comprehension of this complex journey, "Stroke Recovery Roadmap" is your compass, your guide, and your confidant.

This guide is a versatile resource, much like the recovery journey itself. While it can certainly be devoured from cover to cover, it is equally designed to cater to your immediate needs and concerns. Each chapter is a self-contained reservoir of knowledge, empowering you to explore facets of stroke recovery that resonate most deeply with your current circumstances.

Between these pages, you will unearth a treasure trove of information spanning a vast spectrum of topics. Whether your quest is for insights into recognizing the signs and symptoms of a stroke, guidance on physical rehabilitation exercises, comprehension of the emotional labyrinth that may unfurl, or strategies for seamlessly reestablishing daily life post-stroke, this guide offers a multifaceted arsenal of knowledge. Personal narratives, expert perspectives, and pragmatic counsel await you, all with a single, overarching purpose: to provide not only information but also authentic support, encouragement, and a profound sense of direction.

So, with this introduction as our embarkation point, let us commence this voyage of healing and discovery together. "Stroke Recovery Roadmap" is not just a book; it is a map, a fellow traveler, and a ray of hope. May the pages that follow serve as a wellspring of empowerment, inspiration, and enlightenment as we traverse the intricate path toward recovery after stroke.

CHAPTER ONE: UNDERSTANDING STROKE

In this foundational chapter, we delve deep into the intricate world of strokes. We explore the essence of what a stroke truly is, uncovering its diverse forms and the risk factors that weave its narrative. But beyond the clinical, we navigate the human aspect, decoding the subtle warning signs and symptoms that demand our attention. It's a journey into the heart of stroke awareness, a compass for understanding the uncharted terrain of this condition that touches so many lives.

What is a Stroke?

A stroke, often referred to as a cerebrovascular event, stands as one of the most intricate and potentially life-altering medical conditions. At its core, it represents a sudden and profound disruption of the normal blood flow to the brain. This interruption is akin to a sudden power outage in a bustling city, with dire consequences that ripple throughout the brain's intricate network of cells and circuits.

There are two primary categories into which strokes fall, each governed by its own unique set of circumstances: ischemic strokes and hemorrhagic strokes.

Ischemic Strokes: These strokes are the most prevalent and occur when a cerebral blood vessel becomes obstructed or blocked. This blockage can arise from various sources, including blood clots, emboli, or the gradual buildup of atherosclerotic plaque within the arteries. The result is that a vital channel for the delivery of oxygen and nutrients to a particular region of the brain becomes obstructed, leading to a cascade of events that disrupt neural function. As this area of the brain is starved of its life-sustaining resources, neurons begin to falter and, if the blood flow remains compromised, can ultimately succumb. This phenomenon, known as cerebral infarction, underpins the plethora of symptoms that are commonly associated with ischemic strokes.

Hemorrhagic Strokes: While less frequent than ischemic strokes, hemorrhagic strokes are equally formidable. These strokes occur when a blood vessel within the brain experiences a rupture, giving rise to bleeding into the adjacent neural tissue. This sudden and uncontrolled hemorrhage initiates the formation of a hematoma—an accumulation of blood that can exert pressure on the surrounding brain structures. Unlike ischemic strokes, where the disruption originates from an insufficient supply of blood, hemorrhagic strokes unleash the destructive potential of an excessive blood presence within the cranial cavity. This can lead to the elevation of intracranial pressure, further compounding brain injury.

The repercussions of brain damage resulting from a stroke are intricate and multi-faceted, contingent upon numerous factors. The specific location within the brain where damage occurs plays a pivotal role, as different regions govern distinct functions. For instance, damage to the motor cortex may result in paralysis or weakness on one side of the body—a condition known as hemiparesis or hemiplegia. Sensory disturbances, such as numbness or tingling, may also manifest. Language and communication challenges, in the form of aphasia, can become apparent, alongside cognitive deficits encompassing memory impairment, difficulties with reasoning, and alterations in perception.

Emotional challenges are frequently intertwined with stroke-related physical and cognitive impairments. Depression, anxiety, and emotional lability often emerge, affecting both the individual who has experienced the stroke and their loved ones.

It is essential to appreciate the intricate nature of strokes, their subtypes, and the potential consequences of brain damage. Such understanding is not merely academic; it is instrumental in both prevention and effective management. Swift recognition of warning signs, timely medical intervention, and comprehensive rehabilitation programs are pivotal in mitigating the long-term impact of a stroke. Stroke awareness and education are foundational in empowering individuals, caregivers, and healthcare providers to recognize symptoms promptly, take swift action, and provide essential support in the critical hours and days following a stroke.

Types of Strokes

Within the intricate landscape of stroke pathology, two primary categories emerge, each characterized by distinct etiologies, risk factors, and clinical presentations: ischemic strokes and hemorrhagic strokes. Delving deeper into these divergent strokes allows us to appreciate the intricate web of factors that contribute to their onset and the nuanced consequences they entail.

Ischemic Strokes

Causes and Mechanisms: Ischemic strokes, comprising approximately 85% of all stroke cases, occur when a cerebral blood vessel becomes obstructed or occluded, impeding the flow of blood to a specific area of the brain. Several underlying conditions can precipitate this blockage, each with its own set of risk factors. The most common culprits include:

1. **Thrombotic Stroke**: This subtype arises from the formation of a blood clot (thrombus) within a cerebral artery, often in association with atherosclerosis—a condition characterized by the buildup of plaque within the arteries. Risk factors for thrombotic strokes encompass hypertension, diabetes, high cholesterol, smoking, and a family history of stroke.

2. **Embolic Stroke**: In cases of embolic strokes, an embolus—a clot or debris formed elsewhere in the body—travels through the bloodstream until it lodges in a cerebral artery, obstructing blood flow to the brain. Common sources of emboli include the heart (in conditions like atrial fibrillation), carotid arteries, or other large vessels. Risk factors include heart disease, atrial fibrillation, previous strokes, and certain medical procedures that can dislodge emboli.

Clinical Presentation: Ischemic strokes can manifest as a spectrum of symptoms, contingent upon the location and size of the affected brain region. Common symptoms include sudden weakness or paralysis of one side of the body (hemiparesis or hemiplegia), slurred speech or difficulty speaking (aphasia), visual disturbances, and cognitive impairments, such as memory loss or difficulty with reasoning.

Hemorrhagic Strokes

Causes and Mechanisms: Hemorrhagic strokes, while less prevalent than their ischemic counterparts, pose equally formidable challenges. They arise from the rupture of a blood vessel within the brain, leading to bleeding into the surrounding neural tissue. The two primary subtypes of hemorrhagic strokes are intracerebral hemorrhage and subarachnoid hemorrhage, each with its distinct causes and risk factors:

1. **Intracerebral Hemorrhage**: This form of hemorrhagic stroke occurs when a small blood vessel within the brain ruptures, releasing blood into the surrounding brain tissue. Chronic hypertension stands as a dominant risk factor, as prolonged high blood pressure can weaken vessel walls over time, making them more susceptible to rupture. Other contributors include the use of blood-thinning medications, structural abnormalities like arteriovenous malformations (AVMs), and substance abuse.

2. **Subarachnoid Hemorrhage**: Subarachnoid hemorrhages involve bleeding into the space between the brain and the protective membranes that envelop it, known as the subarachnoid space. The most common cause is the rupture of an intracranial aneurysm—a weakened, balloon-like bulge in a blood vessel. Risk factors for subarachnoid hemorrhage include a family history of aneurysms, smoking, hypertension, and certain congenital conditions that predispose individuals to aneurysm formation.

Clinical Presentation: Hemorrhagic strokes often present with a sudden, severe headache, often described as the "worst headache of my life." Other symptoms may include nausea, vomiting, altered consciousness, and neurological deficits corresponding to the site of bleeding.

Appreciating the nuances and complexities of ischemic and hemorrhagic strokes, along with their associated risk factors, empowers individuals, healthcare providers, and caregivers with the knowledge needed for early recognition, intervention, and preventive measures. Stroke awareness, risk factor management, and swift medical attention remain vital components in mitigating the devastating impact of these neurological emergencies.

Risk Factors

A profound understanding of the intricate landscape of risk factors is essential. These factors encompass a diverse array of conditions and behaviors that significantly influence an individual's susceptibility to experiencing a stroke. They can be broadly categorized into two groups: non-modifiable, representing inherent traits or conditions that cannot be altered, and modifiable, indicating those factors where lifestyle changes and medical interventions can effectively mitigate risk.

An in-depth exploration of these risk factors illuminates the complex interplay between genetics, behavior, and healthcare, ultimately paving the way for enhanced stroke prevention strategies and overall health improvement.

Non-Modifiable Risk Factors

1. **Age**: Advanced age stands as one of the most potent non-modifiable risk factors for stroke. As individuals grow older, their risk of stroke escalates significantly. The majority of strokes occur in individuals aged 65 and older, underscoring the importance of age as a determinant.

2. **Gender**: While strokes can affect individuals of any gender, certain gender-specific risk factors exist. For instance, women tend to live longer than men, increasing their lifetime risk. Moreover, some stroke risk factors, such as birth control pill use and complications during pregnancy, are exclusive to women, necessitating gender-tailored preventive measures.

3. **Family History**: A familial predisposition to stroke or transient ischemic attacks (TIAs) can elevate an individual's risk. This genetic propensity underscores the role of inherited traits and shared environmental factors in stroke vulnerability.

4. **Race and Ethnicity**: Epidemiological data has consistently shown that certain racial and ethnic groups, including African Americans, Hispanics, and specific Asian populations, confront a heightened risk of stroke. The multifaceted nature of this elevated risk can be attributed to a combination of genetic factors, socio-economic disparities, and disparities in healthcare

access and quality. Understanding these disparities is integral to devising targeted preventive strategies for at-risk populations.

Modifiable Risk Factors

1. **Hypertension (High Blood Pressure)**: Elevated blood pressure ranks among the most influential modifiable risk factors for stroke. The effective management of blood pressure through lifestyle changes and medications can substantially reduce the risk of stroke. Blood pressure control represents a cornerstone of stroke prevention.

2. **Smoking**: Tobacco use, whether through smoking or exposure to secondhand smoke, is a potent and entirely modifiable risk factor. The act of quitting smoking leads to a significant reduction in the risk of stroke over time, highlighting the pivotal role of behavioral change in stroke prevention.

3. **Diabetes**: Uncontrolled diabetes can lead to vascular damage and heightened stroke risk. The rigorous management of diabetes, encompassing blood sugar control and regular monitoring, is pivotal in risk reduction.

4. **High Cholesterol**: Elevated levels of cholesterol, notably low-density lipoprotein (LDL) cholesterol, can contribute to atherosclerosis—a cornerstone in ischemic stroke pathology.

Dietary modifications, medication regimens, and lifestyle changes are instrumental in managing cholesterol levels.

5. **Physical Inactivity**: A sedentary lifestyle and a lack of regular exercise are key drivers of obesity and other risk factors, including hypertension and diabetes. The engagement in regular physical activity, alongside the adoption of an active lifestyle, plays a crucial role in risk mitigation.

6. **Obesity**: Excessive body weight, particularly when concentrated around the abdomen, is intricately linked to an increased risk of stroke. The maintenance of a healthy weight through dietary adjustments, physical activity, and behavioral modifications is a fundamental component of stroke prevention.

7. **Dietary Factors**: Dietary habits significantly influence stroke risk. A diet rich in saturated fats, excessive sodium (salt) intake, and the consumption of processed foods can contribute to the development of hypertension, high cholesterol, and obesity. Conversely, a balanced diet characterized by the consumption of fruits, vegetables, whole grains, lean proteins, and limited sodium intake can substantially lower stroke risk.

8. **Alcohol Consumption**: Excessive alcohol intake can lead to the elevation of blood pressure and contribute to heart rhythm abnormalities, both of which heighten stroke risk. Limiting

alcohol consumption represents a modifiable behavior that significantly influences risk.

9. **Atrial Fibrillation (AFib)**: This heart rhythm disorder can lead to the formation of blood clots in the heart, which may subsequently travel to the brain and cause a stroke. Managing AFib with medication, lifestyle adjustments, and medical monitoring is essential for risk reduction.

10. **Drug Abuse**: Illicit drug use, particularly substances like cocaine and amphetamines, has been associated with an elevated risk of stroke. The recognition of drug abuse as a modifiable risk factor necessitates seeking help to overcome addiction and prevent associated medical consequences.

11. **Sleep Apnea**: Untreated sleep apnea, characterized by disrupted breathing during sleep, is increasingly recognized as a modifiable risk factor for stroke. The management of sleep apnea through interventions such as continuous positive airway pressure (CPAP) therapy can mitigate this risk.

12. **Stress and Mental Health**: Chronic stress and specific mental health conditions, including depression, have been linked to an increased risk of stroke. Behavioral interventions, stress management techniques, and access to mental health support systems play an instrumental role in risk reduction.

The recognition and differentiation between modifiable and non-modifiable stroke risk factors underscore the significance of proactive risk factor management. Lifestyle modifications, medication adherence, and regular healthcare assessments collectively empower individuals to mitigate their risk of stroke while simultaneously improving their overall well-being.

Additionally, the synergy between risk factor management and stroke awareness empowers individuals to make informed choices about their health and take proactive steps in reducing their vulnerability to this often preventable medical condition. Stroke prevention is a multifaceted endeavor that hinges on comprehensive risk factor management, early recognition of symptoms, and a commitment to proactive healthcare.

Warning Signs and Symptoms

Timely response to the warning signs and symptoms of a stroke can be the decisive factor in preventing severe and lasting consequences. Strokes can manifest in various ways, but a thorough understanding of the common indicators, along with the mnemonic FAST (Face, Arms, Speech, Time), is essential for recognizing a stroke quickly and taking appropriate action.

Common Stroke Symptoms

1. **Sudden Numbness or Weakness**: One of the most recognizable signs of a stroke is the abrupt onset of numbness or weakness, typically occurring on one side of the body. This can manifest as a sudden inability to move or control an arm, leg, or facial muscles on one side.

2. **Difficulty Speaking or Understanding Speech**: Stroke can significantly impact language abilities. Individuals experiencing a stroke may exhibit slurred speech, difficulty forming words, or an inability to comprehend spoken language. These communication challenges are often pronounced and alarming.

3. **Confusion and Disorientation**: A stroke can lead to sudden confusion or disorientation. Affected individuals may find it challenging to grasp their surroundings, determine the current time, or comprehend the situation they are in.

4. **Severe Headache**: A sudden, severe headache, often described as "the worst headache of my life," can be indicative of a hemorrhagic stroke. This type of stroke involves bleeding within the brain, and the accompanying headache is typically intense and different from routine headaches. It may be accompanied by other neurological symptoms.

5. **Trouble Walking or Maintaining Balance**: A stroke can disrupt coordination and balance, making it difficult for individuals to walk steadily or stand upright. Some may stagger, lose their balance, or experience a profound lack of coordination.

6. **Visual Disturbances**: Sudden alterations in vision are potential warning signs of a stroke. These may include blurred vision, double vision, or a complete loss of vision in one or both eyes. Visual disturbances may be temporary or persistent.

7. **Dizziness and Vertigo**: Sudden dizziness, a spinning sensation (vertigo), or a profound loss of balance can occur during a stroke. These symptoms can be disorienting and disconcerting.

The FAST Acronym for Stroke Recognition

The FAST acronym is a valuable mnemonic to quickly assess and recognize potential stroke symptoms:

- **F for Face**: Instruct the individual to display a smile. A drooping or uneven smile, particularly if one side of the face appears to sag, can be a sign of a stroke.

- **A for Arms**: Instruct the person to raise both arms. If one arm drifts downward or is noticeably weaker than the other, it may indicate a stroke.

- **S for Speech**: Have the person repeat a simple sentence. Slurred speech, difficulty in pronouncing words, or the inability to speak coherently can be indicative of a stroke.

- **T for Time**: Time is of the essence in stroke management. If you observe any of these signs or symptoms in yourself or someone else, call emergency services immediately. Rapid medical intervention can significantly improve the outcome of a stroke.

It is crucial to underscore that strokes can manifest differently in each individual, and not all warning signs may be evident. Additionally, stroke symptoms can evolve or change rapidly. Recognizing any of these signs, even if they are transient or seem to resolve, warrants immediate medical attention.

Every second counts in the management of a stroke, and timely intervention can make a substantial difference in the extent of recovery and long-term outcomes. Stroke awareness, coupled with a commitment to acting swiftly, is a vital component of stroke prevention and care. In stroke care, time lost is indeed brain lost, making early recognition and action the ultimate keys to positive outcomes.

CHAPTER TWO: IMMEDIATE POST-STROKE CARE

In the wake of a stroke, the immediate hours that follow are profoundly consequential. This chapter delves into the crucial aspects of post-stroke care, encompassing the first critical hours, hospitalization, and the array of medical treatments that may be administered. We explore the multidisciplinary teams and specialists integral to stroke recovery, emphasizing the collaborative effort required for comprehensive rehabilitation. Setting realistic expectations is also paramount; this chapter guides you in understanding the complexities of stroke recovery while fostering hope and determination.

The First Hours After a Stroke

The immediate hours following the onset of a stroke are nothing short of critical. During this time, the urgency of prompt medical intervention becomes abundantly clear, as each passing moment plays a decisive role in determining the extent of brain damage and, consequently, the long-term prognosis for the stroke survivor. To grasp the gravity of this phase in stroke care, it is imperative to comprehend the vital significance of time and to gain insight into the comprehensive evaluation that unfolds when a stroke patient arrives at the hospital.

The Importance of Time

At the heart of stroke care lies an inescapable truth—the relentless march of time. Stroke is a dynamic, time-sensitive medical emergency where every second matters. The urgency stems from the fundamental nature of strokes, which typically occur when there is a disruption in the blood supply to a part of the brain. This interruption leads to the dire consequences of oxygen and nutrient deprivation, ultimately culminating in the death of brain cells.

Immediate medical attention is paramount for two primary reasons, both underscored by the imperative of time:

1. **Minimizing Brain Damage**: Timely intervention is akin to unlocking a vital portal to stroke recovery. It can help swiftly restore blood flow to the affected part of the brain, thereby potentially curtailing the extent of brain tissue damage. This critical step serves as a pivotal determinant in shaping the degree of disability and impairment that an individual may experience in the aftermath of a stroke.

2. **Administering Treatment**: In specific cases, particularly those involving ischemic strokes (which result from the blockage of a blood vessel supplying the brain), treatment options exist that can substantially mitigate the impact of the stroke. These treatments may encompass the use of clot-dissolving medications, such as tissue plasminogen activator (tPA), or

mechanical thrombectomy—a procedure designed to physically remove the clot obstructing the blood vessel. However, the effectiveness of these treatments hinges on their administration within precise timeframes following the onset of symptoms. Delayed presentation to the hospital can compromise the eligibility for these interventions or diminish their efficacy, underscoring the irreplaceable value of time.

The Initial Evaluation at the Hospital

When a stroke patient arrives at the hospital, a well-orchestrated sequence of actions unfolds with remarkable efficiency. This initial evaluation is characterized by a systematic and comprehensive approach aimed at rapidly assessing the patient's condition, pinpointing the type of stroke, and determining the most suitable course of action. ,

Key components of this evaluation encompass:

1. **Rapid Assessment of Vital Signs**: The foremost priority is to assess the patient's vital signs, encompassing parameters like blood pressure, heart rate, and oxygen saturation levels. Ensuring the patient's physiological stability lays the foundation for subsequent interventions.

2. **Focused Neurological Examination**: A meticulous neurological examination is conducted to gauge the patient's

level of consciousness, responsiveness, and the presence of any neurological deficits. This assessment serves as a crucial linchpin in discerning the type and severity of the stroke, thereby guiding subsequent decisions.

3. **Imaging Studies**: Rapid brain imaging is imperative in the differentiation between ischemic and hemorrhagic strokes. A non-contrast CT scan, frequently employed for this purpose, plays a pivotal role in elucidating the nature of the stroke and facilitating treatment decisions.

4. **Blood Tests**: Comprehensive blood tests are performed to assess various parameters, including blood glucose levels and coagulation profiles. These tests serve to rule out alternative causes of stroke-like symptoms and provide critical insights into the patient's overall health.

5. **Treatment Decisions**: Armed with the results of the evaluation, healthcare providers embark on the journey of making nuanced treatment decisions. These decisions may encompass the initiation of clot-dissolving medications (when applicable), the careful management of blood pressure, and the diligent addressing of any coexisting medical conditions that may complicate stroke care.

The orchestration of this evaluation is facilitated by the presence of specialized stroke teams and established protocols within hospital settings. These teams, comprising healthcare professionals adept at stroke care, work in harmony to streamline the assessment and treatment process, ensuring that each precious minute is harnessed to the patient's advantage. In the journey through the first hours after a stroke, it becomes unequivocally clear that time is the most precious commodity. These initial hours, often fraught with uncertainty and anxiety, hold the key to unlocking the potential for optimal recovery and rehabilitation.

Understanding the urgency of seeking immediate medical attention when stroke symptoms manifest, coupled with insights into the initial hospital evaluation process, empowers individuals and their caregivers to navigate this critical phase with confidence. The first hours after a stroke embody a race—a race against brain damage—where time lost is indeed brain lost, and where swift and informed action emerges as the ultimate imperative.

Hospitalization and Medical Treatment

When a patient is admitted to the hospital with symptoms of a stroke, it is imperative to provide meticulous and comprehensive medical treatment to minimize brain damage and optimize the chances of a successful recovery. This section will delve into the typical treatments that stroke patients receive in a hospital setting, including thrombolytic therapy (clot-busting drugs), surgical interventions, and vigilant monitoring for complications.

Initial Assessment and Stabilization

Upon admission, medical professionals embark on a systematic evaluation of the patient's medical history, including any pre-existing medical conditions and medications. This comprehensive exploration seeks to uncover potential risk factors and prior health issues that may influence the course of treatment.

Advanced imaging tests such as CT (Computed Tomography) scans or MRI (Magnetic Resonance Imaging) scans are promptly conducted to discern the type and location of the stroke (whether it is ischemic or hemorrhagic) and to rule out alternative diagnoses. These images serve as the foundation for treatment decisions and provide critical insights into the extent of brain damage.

Vital signs are rigorously monitored, including blood pressure, heart rate, respiratory rate, and oxygen saturation. Immediate interventions are initiated to stabilize the patient's condition. This includes ensuring an adequate oxygen supply through supplemental oxygen or mechanical ventilation, controlling elevated blood pressure to prevent further damage, and addressing any respiratory issues, such as airway management or mechanical ventilation if necessary.

Thrombolytic Therapy

If the stroke is determined to be of ischemic origin (caused by a blood clot) and the patient presents within a specific time window (typically within 4.5 hours of symptom onset), they may be eligible for thrombolytic therapy.

Thrombolytic drugs, most commonly tissue plasminogen activator (tPA), are administered intravenously. These drugs work by dissolving the clot obstructing the affected blood vessel, thereby restoring blood flow to the deprived area of the brain. The process of administering tPA is a delicate balance between the potential benefits of clot dissolution and the inherent risks, particularly the potential for bleeding complications.

Thrombolytic therapy carries inherent risks, including the potential for bleeding, especially if the patient has recently undergone surgery, has a history of bleeding disorders, or presents with severe hypertension. Consequently, meticulous monitoring is crucial during and after the administration of these drugs. Regular assessments of vital signs and neurological status are performed, and imaging studies may be repeated to assess treatment efficacy and evaluate for complications.

Mechanical Thrombectomy

In cases where the clot is sizable, or thrombolytic therapy alone is ineffective, a mechanical thrombectomy may be considered. This procedure is often performed by interventional radiologists or neurosurgeons and involves the insertion of a catheter into the affected blood vessel.

The catheter is equipped with specialized devices, such as stent retrievers or aspiration systems, which are used to physically remove or retrieve the clot. The success of mechanical thrombectomy largely depends on factors such as the clot's size, location, and the timeliness of the intervention.

While mechanical thrombectomy can be highly effective in restoring blood flow to the brain, it is not without risks. Complications, such as vessel injury or clot fragmentation, may arise during the procedure, necessitating meticulous monitoring and swift interventions to address any adverse events.

Blood Pressure Management

Elevated blood pressure is a common risk factor for stroke and can exacerbate the condition. Healthcare providers employ various strategies to manage blood pressure while avoiding hypotension (abnormally low blood pressure).

Medications may be administered, and intravenous infusions carefully titrated to achieve optimal blood pressure levels. The delicate balance between reducing blood pressure to prevent further damage and maintaining adequate cerebral perfusion is a central consideration in stroke care.

Monitoring for Complications

Stroke patients are subjected to meticulous and continuous monitoring throughout their hospital stay to detect and promptly manage potential complications. This vigilant oversight extends beyond the acute phase of treatment to encompass the entire period of hospitalization.

Common complications include brain swelling (edema), infections, pneumonia, and the formation of blood clots, which may lead to deep vein thrombosis or pulmonary embolism. Timely interventions such as diuretics to reduce cerebral edema, antibiotics to treat infections, and blood-thinning medications to prevent clot formation may be prescribed as necessary.

Rehabilitation and Post-Stroke Care Planning

Following the acute phase of treatment, stroke patients often require an extended period of rehabilitation to regain lost functions and improve their overall quality of life. Rehabilitation is a multifaceted approach encompassing various therapies and interventions.

Physical therapy aims to enhance motor skills, improve mobility, and strengthen weakened muscles. Occupational therapy focuses on aiding patients to regain independence in activities of daily living, such as dressing, grooming, and cooking. Speech therapy addresses communication difficulties and helps patients overcome swallowing challenges. Additionally, psychological support is integral to managing emotional and cognitive challenges that may arise as a result of the stroke.

A multidisciplinary team of healthcare professionals, including physiatrists, physical therapists, occupational therapists, speech-language pathologists, and psychologists, collaborates to develop a personalized care plan tailored to each patient's specific needs and goals. The duration and intensity of rehabilitation vary depending on the severity of the stroke and the individual's progress.

Prevention and Education

Hospitalization provides an ideal opportunity for healthcare professionals to educate both patients and their families about stroke risk factors, prevention strategies, and lifestyle modifications. Education is a proactive approach to reducing the risk of recurrent strokes and promoting overall health and well-being.

Discharge planning is a critical component of care, ensuring that patients receive appropriate follow-up care and ongoing support in the post-hospitalization phase. This comprehensive approach includes medication management, dietary recommendations, and lifestyle modifications such as smoking cessation, dietary adjustments, increased physical activity, and stress management strategies.

In summary, hospitalization and medical treatment for stroke patients involve an exhaustive and highly coordinated approach that spans the spectrum from initial assessment and stabilization to advanced therapies, vigilant monitoring, rehabilitation, and prevention. Early diagnosis, prompt administration of clot-dissolving therapies or mechanical thrombectomy when indicated, meticulous monitoring for complications, and a strong emphasis on rehabilitation and education all contribute to optimizing outcomes and improving the patient's chances of recovery.

Stroke care is a complex and multifaceted endeavor that requires the expertise of a dedicated team of healthcare professionals working in concert to provide the highest level of care and support to stroke patients and their families.

Rehabilitation Teams and Specialists

Stroke rehabilitation is a multidimensional journey, a voyage through which a coordinated team of healthcare professionals guides patients with unwavering dedication. In this chapter, we will elucidate the key members of the stroke rehabilitation team, each a crucial pillar in the recovery process. Their collaborative efforts culminate in the creation of a customized recovery plan that paves the way for renewed hope and restored functionality.

Neurologists: The Captains of Stroke Care

Neurologists serve as the navigators of the stroke rehabilitation journey. They are specialized physicians with expertise in the diagnosis and treatment of neurological disorders, including stroke. Their role begins in the acute phase of stroke care, where they play a pivotal role in determining the type and severity of the stroke, often through imaging studies such as CT scans or MRIs.

In the rehabilitation phase, neurologists continue to be central figures. They assess the patient's neurological deficits, track progress, and adjust treatment plans as needed. Their insights into the neurological intricacies of stroke ensure that the rehabilitation process is tailored to the patient's specific needs.

Physical Therapists: Masters of Mobility

Physical therapists are the architects of mobility and strength. They work closely with stroke patients to restore physical functionality, such as walking, balance, and muscle strength. A customized exercise regimen is crafted to address the patient's specific deficits and goals.

During rehabilitation, physical therapists employ various techniques and exercises to improve mobility. These may include gait training, exercises to enhance limb coordination, and strategies to increase endurance. The overarching objective is to help patients regain their independence in activities of daily living.

Occupational Therapists: Rebuilding Daily Living Skills

Occupational therapists focus on the intricate tapestry of daily living activities. They evaluate the patient's ability to perform essential tasks, such as dressing, grooming, cooking, and managing household chores. Occupational therapists then work collaboratively with patients to relearn these skills and adapt to any lasting physical or cognitive challenges.

The rehabilitation process often involves the use of adaptive equipment or techniques tailored to the patient's unique needs. Occupational therapists are instrumental in ensuring that stroke survivors can regain independence and resume their roles within their families and communities.

Speech-Language Pathologists: Guardians of Communication and Swallowing

Stroke can significantly impact communication and swallowing abilities. Speech-language pathologists step into this critical realm, evaluating and treating speech, language, cognition, and swallowing disorders. They are trained to identify and address deficits in speech articulation, language comprehension and expression, and cognitive impairments related to stroke.

In cases where stroke has caused dysphagia or swallowing difficulties, speech-language pathologists work to assess and manage this condition. They employ strategies and exercises to improve swallowing safety and minimize the risk of aspiration pneumonia, a common concern in stroke survivors.

Rehabilitation Nurses: The Compassionate Caregivers

Rehabilitation nurses serve as compassionate caregivers in the rehabilitation team. They provide round-the-clock care, monitor patients' vital signs, administer medications, and coordinate various aspects of the patient's rehabilitation plan. Their role extends beyond medical care; they offer emotional support and encouragement, fostering a positive and nurturing environment for recovery.

Psychologists and Neuropsychologists: Nurturing Emotional Well-Being

Stroke often brings not only physical challenges but also emotional and cognitive changes. Psychologists and neuropsychologists are integral members of the rehabilitation team, addressing the emotional and psychological impact of stroke. They offer counseling, coping strategies, and cognitive rehabilitation to help patients manage emotional distress and cognitive deficits.

Social Workers and Case Managers: The Advocates of Support

Social workers and case managers play pivotal roles in helping stroke survivors navigate the complex web of healthcare and social services. They assist in coordinating care, connecting patients with community resources, and addressing practical concerns related to housing, insurance, and financial support. Their advocacy ensures that patients receive comprehensive support beyond the walls of the rehabilitation facility.

The Collaborative Symphony of Rehabilitation

Collaboration is the cornerstone of stroke rehabilitation. These specialists work in unison, sharing insights and observations to craft a personalized recovery plan. Regular team meetings allow for the alignment of goals, tracking progress, and adjusting interventions as needed.

The stroke rehabilitation team considers the patient's unique strengths, weaknesses, and aspirations when tailoring the recovery plan. This individualized approach ensures that each patient receives the care and support required to maximize their potential for recovery.

In summary, stroke rehabilitation is a collaborative effort orchestrated by a multidisciplinary team of specialists. Neurologists, physical therapists, occupational therapists, speech-language pathologists, and other healthcare professionals come together to guide stroke survivors along the path to recovery. Their expertise, dedication, and coordinated efforts empower patients to rebuild their lives and rekindle hope in the aftermath of a stroke.

Setting Realistic Expectations

The journey of stroke recovery is as much a psychological odyssey as it is a physical one. In this section, we delve deep into the complex emotional terrain that stroke survivors traverse, highlighting the paramount importance of setting achievable short-term and long-term recovery goals. This section aims to provide comprehensive guidance on embracing patience and perseverance as unwavering companions on the path to recovery.

The Emotional Landscape of Stroke Recovery

A stroke is a life-altering event, that shakes the very foundations of an individual's existence. It ushers in a torrent of emotions that can range from shock and fear to anger, sadness, and frustration. The suddenness of the stroke and its often unforeseen consequences can be emotionally overwhelming.

The emotional impact extends its reach, touching not just the survivor but also reverberating through the lives of family members and caregivers. Loved ones grapple with adjusting to new roles and responsibilities, witnessing the challenges faced by their dear ones, and navigating the uncertainties that shroud the recovery journey.

The Invaluable Role of Realistic Expectations

Amid this emotional turbulence, setting realistic expectations emerges as an invaluable guiding light. While it is entirely natural to yearn for a swift return to the life that existed before the stroke, the reality of stroke recovery is often a gradual process, marked by incremental milestones interspersed with occasional setbacks.

Short-term Recovery Goals: The Building Blocks of Hope

Short-term recovery goals serve as the foundational building blocks upon which the edifice of rehabilitation stands. They are the practical, achievable objectives that encompass regaining the ability to perform daily tasks—perhaps dressing independently or taking a few unassisted steps. These goals are specific, measurable, and realistically attainable within a relatively short timeframe.

The significance of celebrating these small victories cannot be overstated. Each accomplishment signifies progress, serves as a morale booster, and instills a profound sense of accomplishment. Recognizing and acknowledging these achievements fosters a positive mindset and acts as a powerful antidote against the creeping sense of frustration or impatience that may sometimes cloud the recovery journey.

Long-term Recovery Goals: The Summits in the Distance

Long-term recovery goals, on the other hand, are the summits that loom in the distance, casting a far-reaching vision. These are the aspirations that may involve reclaiming full independence, returning to work, or achieving the highest possible level of functionality. They often demand sustained effort, time, and unwavering dedication.

Setting these long-term goals provides a sense of direction and purpose. They are the guiding stars on the recovery horizon, illuminating the path forward. However, it is imperative to recognize that the journey toward these goals may not be a linear trajectory. There may be plateaus where progress seems stagnant, and, at times, there might even be temporary setbacks. The key lies in maintaining resilience and an unwavering commitment to the overarching vision of recovery.

The Virtues of Patience and Perseverance

Patience, the steady companion of recovery, is a virtue that assumes unparalleled significance. It is the recognition that healing is a journey that unfolds in its own time, often defying the impatience that yearns for immediate results. Patience is the ability to frame setbacks as stepping stones to progress, to learn from them rather than being disheartened by them.

Perseverance, likewise, stands as the stalwart resolve to persist in the face of challenges. It is the unwavering determination to continue the struggle, to remain undaunted by the obstacles that occasionally block the path. Perseverance acknowledges that every effort, no matter how seemingly small, contributes to the larger tapestry of recovery.

The Power of Support and Resources

The emotional challenges of setting realistic expectations and navigating the recovery landscape can be substantially eased through the embrace of a robust support network. Connecting with support groups, counselors, or therapists can provide a safe haven to share experiences, exchange coping strategies, and find solace in the shared journey of recovery.

Family members and caregivers, too, play a pivotal role in providing the emotional support that is often the bedrock of a survivor's resilience. Open and empathetic communication, the ability to put oneself in the survivor's shoes, and mutual understanding can collectively foster resilience for both the survivor and their support system.

In conclusion, setting realistic expectations is a multifaceted and nuanced aspect of stroke recovery, encompassing short-term and long-term goals. Embracing patience and perseverance as unwavering companions on this journey can empower survivors to navigate the emotional landscape with fortitude and grace. Stroke recovery is not just a testament to the human spirit's resilience; it is a journey filled with hope, possibilities, and the unwavering belief in the power of the human will to overcome adversity.

CHAPTER THREE: THE ROAD TO RECOVERY

In the aftermath of a stroke, the path to recovery unfurls, offering newfound hope and opportunities for rebuilding lives. This chapter embarks on the journey of rehabilitation and healing, exploring a spectrum of vital elements. From the diverse array of rehabilitation and therapy options available to the pivotal role of physical exercises in regaining mobility and strength, it navigates the terrain of speech and language therapy while addressing the intricacies of coping with emotional challenges. Together, these aspects compose the roadmap to recovery, guiding survivors toward renewed vitality and a brighter future.

Rehabilitation and Therapy Options

Stroke recovery is a dynamic journey characterized by distinct phases of rehabilitation, each with its unique focus, duration, and contributions to the overall path of recovery. In this comprehensive exploration, we delve into these phases in depth, shedding light on their benefits and how they play integral roles in the comprehensive stroke recovery process.

Acute Rehabilitation

Benefits: Acute rehabilitation is the initial phase of stroke recovery and typically commences shortly after the stroke event, often within the hospital setting. Its primary aim is to address the immediate needs of stroke survivors. This phase is crucial for stabilizing the patient's medical condition, preventing complications, and initiating early therapeutic interventions.

Contributions: During the acute rehabilitation phase, a multidisciplinary rehabilitation team, comprising physiatrists, physical therapists, occupational therapists, and speech-language pathologists, among others, collaborates to assess the patient's functional abilities and identify deficits. Immediate therapeutic interventions are initiated to mitigate impairment and disability. Acute rehabilitation sets the foundation for the subsequent phases of recovery by kickstarting the rehabilitation journey and laying out the initial goals for improvement.

Subacute Rehabilitation

Benefits: Subacute rehabilitation follows the acute phase and is conducted in specialized rehabilitation facilities or skilled nursing facilities. This phase is particularly valuable for patients who require additional time and support to regain functional independence. Subacute rehabilitation offers a more extended period of focused therapy and care.

Contributions: In the subacute phase, therapy sessions are intensified, focusing on improving mobility, strength, and functional skills. Stroke survivors receive structured rehabilitation interventions tailored to their specific needs. The subacute phase serves as a bridge between acute care and long-term recovery, fostering sustained progress and independence. Patients benefit from a supportive environment conducive to recovery, and the rehabilitation team continues to refine the rehabilitation plan based on evolving goals and capabilities.

Long-term Rehabilitation

Benefits: Long-term rehabilitation encompasses the extended recovery period that follows the acute and subacute phases. It is particularly crucial for stroke survivors with persistent deficits and ongoing rehabilitation needs. Long-term rehabilitation may take place in outpatient settings, at home, or in assisted living facilities.

Contributions: During long-term rehabilitation, the focus shifts to maintaining and enhancing the gains achieved in earlier phases. Therapy sessions continue to target specific deficits and functional challenges. This phase is marked by ongoing rehabilitation, lifestyle adjustments, and the incorporation of learned skills into daily routines. Stroke survivors work closely with rehabilitation professionals to optimize independence and enhance the overall quality of life.

Outpatient Rehabilitation

Benefits: Outpatient rehabilitation offers flexibility for individuals who have transitioned to living at home but still require ongoing therapy and support. It provides a structured environment for continued improvement and adjustment to life after stroke.

Contributions: Outpatient rehabilitation sessions encompass a range of therapies, including physical, occupational, and speech therapy as needed. The emphasis is on fine-tuning skills, addressing specific challenges, and enhancing overall quality of life. This phase encourages self-management and empowers individuals to take an active role in their recovery journey. Stroke survivors benefit from a supportive network of rehabilitation professionals who work collaboratively to achieve individualized goals.

Home-Based Rehabilitation

Benefits: Home-based rehabilitation is tailored to individuals who prefer or require rehabilitation services in the comfort of their own homes. It offers a highly personalized approach, considering the patient's living environment and specific needs.

Contributions: Home-based rehabilitation facilitates therapy sessions that align with the patient's daily routines and challenges within the home setting. Rehabilitation professionals work on improving functional skills, enhancing safety, and supporting the transition to independent living. Stroke survivors and their families actively participate in the rehabilitation process, fostering a sense of empowerment and self-efficacy.

In summary, stroke recovery encompasses a continuum of phases, each with its distinct contributions and significance. Acute rehabilitation addresses immediate needs, subacute rehabilitation provides intensive support, long-term rehabilitation maintains and enhances progress, outpatient rehabilitation fosters independence, and home-based rehabilitation offers a highly personalized approach. The collaborative efforts of rehabilitation professionals across these phases empower stroke survivors to rebuild their lives, regain optimal functionality, and embrace a brighter future post-stroke.

Physical Rehabilitation Exercises

Physical rehabilitation exercises play a pivotal role in stroke recovery, helping individuals regain essential functions, improve mobility, rebuild strength, and enhance coordination. The following comprehensive list of exercises and activities is tailored to stroke survivors, providing step-by-step instructions and essential precautions to ensure safety and effectiveness throughout the rehabilitation process.

Range of Motion Exercises

1. **Neck Stretches:** To improve neck mobility, sit or stand in a comfortable position. Gently tilt your head from side to side, forward and backward, holding each position for 10-15 seconds. Repeat 5-10 times for a soothing stretch that eases tension in the neck muscles.

2. **Shoulder Circles:** Enhance shoulder flexibility and mobility by rotating your shoulders forward and backward in a circular motion. Start with small circles and gradually increase the range of motion as tolerated. Perform 10-15 repetitions in each direction, promoting better shoulder function and reducing stiffness.

Upper Body Strength Exercises

1. **Seated Arm Raises:** While seated in a sturdy chair, hold a lightweight or a water bottle in each hand. Slowly lift your arms forward and upward, then lower them back down. Aim for 2-3 sets of 10-15 repetitions. This exercise strengthens the arms, shoulders, and upper back, improving overall upper body strength.

2. **Wall Push-Ups:** Stand facing a wall, placing your hands on the wall at shoulder height. Lean forward, bending your elbows, and then push back to the starting position. Perform 2-3 sets of 10-

15 repetitions. Wall push-ups help develop chest and arm strength while promoting stability.

Lower Body Strength Exercises

1. **Chair Squats:** Enhance lower body strength by standing in front of a sturdy chair, feet hip-width apart. Slowly lower yourself toward the chair as if you're about to sit down, then stand back up. Repeat 2-3 sets of 10-15 repetitions. Chair squats target the quadriceps, hamstrings, and glutes, supporting improved lower body function.

2. **Leg Raises:** While lying on your back, bend one knee and keep the other leg straight. Lift the straight leg a few inches off the ground and hold for a few seconds before lowering it back down. Switch legs and repeat. Perform 2-3 sets of 10-15 repetitions for each leg. Leg raises focus on strengthening the hip flexors and lower abdominal muscles, facilitating better leg control.

Balance and Coordination Exercises

1. **Single-Leg Stance:** Stand near a sturdy surface, such as a countertop or chair, for support. Lift one foot off the ground and balance on the other for as long as you can comfortably. Switch legs and repeat. Aim for 2-3 sets of 30 seconds to 1 minute on each leg. This exercise enhances balance and stability, crucial for preventing falls.

2. **Tandem Walking:** Improve balance and coordination by taking small steps forward, placing one foot directly in front of the other, similar to walking on a tightrope. Use a support if needed. Execute 2-3 rounds of 10-15 steps in each direction. Tandem walking challenges your balance and refines your gait pattern.

Mobility Exercises

1. **Seated Leg Swings:** While seated on the edge of a chair with your feet flat on the ground, swing one leg forward and backward while keeping your back straight. Repeat with the other leg. Perform 2-3 sets of 10-15 swings for each leg. Seated leg swings promote hip mobility and flexibility.
2. **Standing Hip Circles:** Hold onto a stable surface for support and stand on one leg. Gently make circular motions with the other leg. Perform 2-3 sets of 10-15 circles in each direction for each leg. Standing hip circles enhance hip joint mobility and improve balance.

Precautions

- Always consult with your healthcare provider or physical therapist before initiating any exercise program after a stroke to ensure it is safe and suitable for your condition.
- Begin with exercises that match your current level of strength and mobility, progressively increasing the intensity and complexity as you make progress.

- Execute exercises in a controlled manner to minimize the risk of injury. Ensure the correct body mechanics and posture are upheld continuously.

- Cease any exercise immediately if you experience pain, dizziness, or discomfort, and seek guidance from a healthcare professional.

- Maintain proper hydration and create a comfortable exercise environment to maximize your safety and well-being.

- Consider working closely with a qualified physical therapist who can customize an exercise program to meet your specific needs, monitor your progress, and provide valuable guidance.

- Consistency is paramount in stroke recovery. By regularly engaging in these physical rehabilitation exercises, you can significantly enhance your mobility, strength, and coordination over time, paving the way to a more active and independent lifestyle.

Speech and Language Therapy

Speech and language therapy, a pivotal component of stroke rehabilitation, embarks on a multifaceted journey to rejuvenate and enhance communication skills in individuals who have encountered the profound impact of a stroke. This in-depth exploration of speech therapy unfolds a vast array of exercises, strategies, and techniques, meticulously crafted to not only ameliorate speech articulation and language comprehension but also to facilitate the restoration of effective and meaningful communication.

Speech Articulation Exercises

Speech articulation exercises serve as the cornerstone of speech therapy, diligently designed to refine the clarity and precision of speech sounds. These exercises, intricate in their approach, play a pivotal role in enabling stroke survivors to regain mastery over oral muscle control and overcome the formidable challenges posed by pronunciation impairments. In the realm of speech articulation exercises, the following facets warrant extensive exploration:

1. **Vocalization Mastery:** Commencing with fundamental vocalization exercises, individuals embark on a journey of producing clear and sustained vowel sounds (e.g., "ah," "ee," "oo"). As confidence builds, the transition to consonant-vowel combinations (e.g., "ba," "da," "ka") marks a significant milestone in the path to articulatory excellence.

2. **Precision in Articulation:** Precision becomes the focal point as individuals engage in articulation drills, concentrating on the meticulous pronunciation of specific sounds or words that the stroke has cast under the shadow of challenges. Targeted sounds, such as the elusive "s," the elusive "r," or the intricate "th," beckon individuals toward a realm of articulatory mastery.

3. **Tongue and Lip Mastery:** Strengthening the muscles of the tongue and lips assumes a paramount role in the quest for enhanced speech articulation. Activities encompass a rich tapestry of tongue twisters, lip pursing exercises, tongue elevation drills, and lip trills, each contributing to the orchestration of a harmonious symphony of muscle control.

4. **Intelligibility Unveiled:** The pursuit of intelligibility enhancement entails the development of clear and deliberate speech patterns, where emphasis is placed not just on diction but also on the art of word and phrase separation. As individuals progress, they artfully increase the cadence of their speech while preserving the sanctity of clarity, ushering in a phase of fluidity in their communication.

Language Comprehension Exercises

Language comprehension exercises form the bedrock of communication recovery. These exercises are instrumental in fortifying the ability to comprehend both spoken and written language, transcending the cognitive challenges that often accompany the aftermath of a stroke. This expansive domain encompasses a mosaic of elements, including:

1. **Auditory Comprehension Odyssey:** Delving into auditory comprehension tasks, individuals engage in an immersive journey of listening to short stories, conversations, or

instructions. The subsequent endeavor involves the art of responding to questions that tether the listener to the core of comprehension. As cognitive prowess flourishes, the complexity of the material unfurls like a blossoming flower.

2. **Literary Landscape:** The literary realm opens its doors as reading comprehension exercises invite individuals to read texts, articles, or books aloud. Discussion ensues, breathing life into the written word. Questions emerge, serving as guides through the labyrinth of understanding.

3. **Lexicon Expansion:** Vocabulary is the tapestry upon which language comprehension thrives. Active participation in vocabulary-building activities unveils the treasure trove of new words. These words, integrated into daily conversations and written expression, serve as bricks in the construction of a linguistic mansion.

4. **Mastery of Instructions:** The ability to follow multi-step instructions serves as both a testament to comprehension and a harbinger of progress. Beginning with elementary tasks, individuals ascend the ladder of complexity, mastering the art of nuanced instructions.

Communication Strategies

Effective communication is an intricate dance that transcends the realms of speech articulation and language comprehension. It encompasses a repertoire of practical communication strategies designed to foster clarity, understanding, and meaningful interaction. Stroke survivors embark on a transformative journey as they master these strategies:

1. **Alternative Communication Avenues:** The expedition of communication often leads to the exploration of alternative paths. Augmentative and alternative communication (AAC) devices, picture boards, and text-to-speech applications emerge as beacons of hope, particularly for those with severe speech impairments.

2. **Contextual Alchemy:** Contextual cues and gestures emerge as the alchemists of understanding, weaving a tapestry of meaning within the fabric of communication. Stroke survivors become adept in the art of deciphering and conveying messages, enveloped by a newfound world of contextual understanding.

3. **Listening as an Art:** Active listening skills are the cornerstone of effective communication. Stroke survivors engage in the art of active listening, a symphony that includes maintaining eye contact, nodding to signify comprehension, and proactively seeking clarification when the mist of uncertainty shrouds the conversation.

4. **The Power of Pacing:** Pacing and well-timed pauses become tools of the trade, strategically incorporated into conversations. These subtle maneuvers grant the gift of time for message

processing and response formulation, ensuring that the essence of communication remains undisturbed.

5. **Visual Reinforcements:** Visual aids, such as written notes or drawings, emerge as powerful allies in the realm of communication. They lend an additional layer of support, fostering comprehension and reinforcing the messages conveyed.

Social Communication Skills

Social communication skills stand as the cornerstone of meaningful interactions, the bridge that connects individuals to the tapestry of social life. Stroke survivors embark on a journey to refine these skills, under the guidance of a seasoned speech-language pathologist (SLP):

1. **Pragmatic Language Mastery:** Pragmatic language skills evolve as stroke survivors delve into the art of appropriate social interaction. Turn-taking in conversations, deciphering the nuances of humor, and maintaining the ebb and flow of conversational topics are essential skills on this odyssey.

2. **The Canvas of Empathy:** Empathy emerges as an integral component of social communication. The stroke survivor learns not only to express emotions authentically but also to empathize with the emotions of others. This transformation elevates the quality of social connections to a profound level.

3. **Social Immersion:** The contours of social interaction come to life as stroke survivors engage in real-life scenarios, participating in communication within the tapestry of group therapy sessions or social gatherings. These opportunities serve as crucibles for honing social communication skills.

4. **Resilience and Emotional Well-being:** Communication challenges, although surmountable, often cast a shadow of frustration or anxiety. Stroke survivors become adept at crafting strategies to navigate these emotional challenges, emerging as resilient champions of their emotional well-being.

Incorporating speech and language therapy into stroke rehabilitation necessitates the forging of a profound partnership between the stroke survivor and a seasoned and compassionate speech-language pathologist (SLP). The voyage unfolds with individualized therapy plans, intricately tailored to address the unique needs and challenges of each individual. Consistency in therapy sessions, unwavering dedication, and the shared commitment of both the stroke survivor and the SLP converge to create a symphony of progress, a testament to the resilience of the human spirit in its quest to rebuild communication and language skills after a stroke.

Coping with Emotional Challenges

A stroke, a sudden and often life-altering event, leaves a profound impact not only on the physical well-being of survivors but also on their emotional landscape. Understanding and effectively managing the emotional aftermath of a stroke are critical aspects of the recovery journey. In this section, we delve deeply into the emotional challenges that frequently accompany stroke, including depression, anxiety, frustration, and grief. Furthermore, we offer detailed insights into these complex emotions, provide an array of coping strategies, introduce relaxation techniques, and guide you in seeking professional mental health support.

Understanding the Emotional Impact

A stroke can evoke a myriad of emotions, both for the survivor and their caregivers. It's essential to acknowledge and comprehend these emotions to effectively address them:

1. **Depression:** Depression is a common emotional response to stroke. It manifests as persistent sadness, loss of interest in previously enjoyable activities, and feelings of hopelessness. Stroke survivors may grapple with the reality of their condition, the challenges of recovery, and the uncertainty of the future, all contributing to depressive symptoms.

2. **Anxiety:** Anxiety often accompanies stroke recovery, characterized by heightened worry and unease. Survivors may experience anxiety due to uncertainties about their health, fear of recurrent strokes, or the stress of adapting to physical and

cognitive changes. It can manifest as restlessness, excessive worry, and even physical symptoms like palpitations.

3. **Frustration and Anger:** Stroke survivors frequently contend with frustration and anger. These emotions stem from the loss of independence, communication difficulties, or the need for ongoing care. Frustration may intensify when faced with the gradual pace of recovery or the inability to perform previously routine tasks.

4. **Grief:** Both the stroke survivor and their loved ones often experience a grieving process. This involves mourning the loss of the life they once knew, with its routines, abilities, and expectations. This grief can be complex and enduring, as adjustments are made to accommodate new realities.

Coping Strategies

Recognizing and addressing these emotions is a pivotal step in the recovery journey. Employing comprehensive coping strategies can significantly help individuals navigate these emotional challenges:

1. **Open Communication:** Encourage open and honest conversations with healthcare providers, family members, and friends. Expressing emotions and concerns can alleviate feelings of isolation and provide crucial emotional support.

2. **Support Groups:** Consider joining stroke support groups or connecting with individuals who have faced similar challenges.

Sharing experiences and coping strategies can foster a sense of camaraderie and understanding, reassuring you that you're not alone in this journey.

3. **Professional Help:** Seeking the assistance of mental health professionals, such as therapists or counselors specializing in stroke recovery, can provide valuable insights and strategies for managing emotions. Therapy offers a safe and confidential space to explore complex feelings and develop coping mechanisms.

4. **Relaxation Techniques:** Practice relaxation techniques like deep breathing exercises, meditation, or progressive muscle relaxation to reduce anxiety and stress. These techniques, which can be learned through therapy or self-help resources, contribute significantly to emotional well-being.

5. **Set Realistic Goals:** Establish both short-term and long-term recovery goals that are achievable. Celebrate even the smallest victories along the way, recognizing that progress in stroke recovery may be gradual but is always meaningful.

6. **Social Engagement:** Stay connected with friends and loved ones. Social support is a powerful buffer against emotional distress. Engaging in enjoyable activities can boost mood and motivation.

7. **Self-Care:** Prioritize self-care by maintaining a healthy lifestyle. Regular physical activity, a balanced diet, and adequate

sleep play crucial roles in positively impacting emotional well-being.

Seeking Professional Mental Health Support

If emotional challenges persist or worsen, seeking professional mental health support is paramount:

1. **Therapy:** Psychotherapy, such as cognitive-behavioral therapy (CBT), can help individuals develop coping strategies, challenge negative thought patterns, and address specific emotional concerns. Therapy offers a structured and supportive environment for emotional healing.

2. **Medication:** In some cases, healthcare providers may prescribe medication to alleviate symptoms of depression or anxiety. Medication should always be prescribed and monitored by a healthcare provider with expertise in mental health and stroke recovery.

3. **Crisis Intervention:** If experiencing intense emotional distress or contemplating self-harm, it's crucial to promptly seek help from emergency services or a crisis hotline. Safety is paramount, and timely intervention can be life-saving.

The Journey Towards Emotional Healing

Coping with emotional challenges is an integral part of the stroke recovery process. It's vital to recognize that these emotions are normal responses to a life-altering event. Seeking help is a sign of strength, and with the right support and strategies, emotional well-being can be nurtured alongside physical recovery.

The emotional journey may be arduous, but it is also an opportunity for growth, resilience, and the discovery of newfound strengths. By acknowledging and addressing these emotional challenges, stroke survivors can find solace, support, and the path to a brighter future, where emotional well-being thrives alongside physical recovery.

CHAPTER FOUR: LIFE AFTER STROKE

As stroke survivors embark on the journey of life after stroke, a new set of challenges and opportunities awaits. This chapter explores the intricacies of navigating daily activities, harnessing adaptive equipment and assistive technology to regain independence, making informed dietary choices to aid recovery, and taking vital steps to prevent secondary strokes. Life after stroke is a path of resilience, adaptation, and empowerment, where survivors and their support networks can work together to reclaim a fulfilling and healthful life.

Navigating Daily Activities

Life after a stroke represents a remarkable journey of rediscovery, especially when it comes to daily activities. Stroke survivors often find themselves grappling with challenges related to self-care, mobility, and home management. Nevertheless, with determination, practical strategies, and the right support system, regaining independence and confidence is not just an aspiration but a tangible goal.

Self-Care:

1. **Personal Hygiene:** Restoring independence in personal hygiene is paramount for stroke survivors. Tasks like bathing, brushing teeth, and dressing can initially pose hurdles. To facilitate these activities, consider installing grab

bars in the bathroom to provide extra stability. A shower chair can offer a secure seating option for those who need it. Adaptive clothing with easy closures, like Velcro or magnetic buttons, simplifies the dressing process. Additionally, explore showerhead extensions and handheld showerheads to enhance accessibility during bathing.

2. **Medication Management:** Consistent medication management is critical. To ensure timely doses, organize medications in pill organizers labeled with days and times. Alternatively, explore medication management apps that send reminders for doses. Seek assistance from a caregiver or healthcare professional if there are concerns about medication adherence. Additionally, consider blister packaging for medications, where doses are pre-packaged in separate compartments, making it easier to track and take medications correctly.

3. **Eating and Drinking:** Dining experiences may require adaptations. For those with limited hand dexterity or mobility, adaptive utensils with easy-to-grip handles can make mealtimes more manageable. Non-slip mats or placemats enhance stability when eating or drinking. Speech therapy may be beneficial for individuals experiencing swallowing difficulties, as therapists can provide guidance

on safer eating techniques and recommend dietary modifications. In addition, explore weighted utensils and cups to counter tremors or shaky hands and ensure more precise control during meals.

Mobility:

1. **Walking:** Gait and mobility often require focused attention. Mobility aids like canes, walkers, or mobility scooters can significantly enhance stability and confidence. Consult with a physical therapist to receive guidance on the most suitable mobility aid. Physical therapy sessions can also address gait and balance issues, helping individuals regain their stride. Consider trying different types of walking aids to find the one that provides the best balance and support for your specific needs.

2. **Transfers:** Transferring between various surfaces, such as chairs, beds, or wheelchairs, can be challenging. Transfer boards or swivel cushions can facilitate smoother transitions. It is essential to practice proper body mechanics to prevent strain or injury during transfers. Occupational therapists can provide personalized training on safe and efficient transfer techniques, taking into account individual strengths and limitations.

3. **Wheelchair Use:** For individuals who rely on wheelchairs, selecting the right wheelchair is paramount. It should be properly fitted to the user's specific needs and body dimensions. Learning to navigate different terrains and obstacles is a valuable skill that can improve mobility and independence. Moreover, explore power wheelchairs if manual propulsion poses difficulties, and ensure the chair's seating and positioning meet comfort and functional requirements.

Home Management:

1. **Household Chores:** Managing household chores necessitates careful planning and adaptation. Prioritize tasks and break them down into manageable segments. Modify the home environment for enhanced accessibility by installing handrails on stairs to provide additional support. In the kitchen, explore adjustable countertops that can be raised or lowered to accommodate sitting or standing positions. Consider a robotic vacuum cleaner to assist with floor cleaning tasks.

2. **Meal Preparation:** Cooking can be simplified with the use of adaptive kitchen tools designed to accommodate varying levels of dexterity. Reachers can assist in accessing items from higher shelves, while elevated countertops provide a

more user-friendly workspace. For added convenience, consider meal delivery services or enlist the support of family members in meal preparation. Invest in kitchen appliances like jar openers, electric can openers, and food processors to reduce manual effort and make meal preparation more manageable.

3. **Safety Measures:** Preventing accidents and falls is a top priority. Remove potential tripping hazards, secure rugs, and ensure adequate lighting throughout the home. Installing smoke alarms and carbon monoxide detectors is crucial for safety and peace of mind. Consider a home safety evaluation by an occupational therapist or a certified aging-in-place specialist to identify and address potential hazards and recommend safety modifications.

4. **Driving:** Many stroke survivors express a desire to resume driving, which requires careful consideration. Consult with a healthcare provider and undergo a thorough driving assessment to determine your fitness for driving. Adaptive driving equipment may be necessary to make driving safe and comfortable. Explore driving rehabilitation programs offered by certified specialists who can assess driving skills, recommend adaptive equipment, and provide training tailored to your specific needs and abilities.

5. **Financial Management:** Simplify financial management tasks by embracing online banking and bill payment services. These platforms provide the convenience of managing finances from home. If the complexity of financial matters feels overwhelming, seek assistance from a trusted family member or a financial advisor to ensure that your financial affairs are in order. Consider setting up automatic payments for recurring bills to ensure they are paid on time, reducing the need for manual financial management.

6. **Social Engagement:** Maintaining social engagement is essential for emotional well-being. Participate in support groups, community events, or hobbies you enjoy to stay connected with others. Arrange for transportation services or explore accessible transportation options to facilitate your participation in social activities. In addition, utilize technology to stay connected with friends and family, and consider joining online support groups to connect with individuals who have similar experiences and challenges.

Remember that progress after a stroke may unfold gradually, and patience is a virtue. Engage in regular physical and occupational therapy sessions to enhance your functional abilities and adapt to the changes in your life. Additionally, involving family members or caregivers in daily activities can provide both practical support and emotional encouragement.

Life after a stroke is indeed a journey of adaptation, where perseverance and the implementation of practical strategies enable stroke survivors to regain their independence and confidence. By systematically addressing self-care, mobility, and home management, stroke survivors can navigate daily activities with increased ease and satisfaction, ultimately enhancing their overall quality of life. The process of regaining independence encompasses a wide range of strategies, adaptations, and technologies that can be tailored to each individual's unique needs and goals, providing a roadmap for a fulfilling life after a stroke.

Adaptive Equipment and Assistive Technology

Emerging triumph after a stroke often hinges on the incorporation of adaptive equipment and assistive technology into one's daily life. These remarkable tools and devices have been meticulously engineered to bridge the gap created by physical or cognitive challenges, facilitating daily activities and elevating the quality of life for stroke survivors. In this in-depth exploration, we embark on a comprehensive journey, uncovering an extensive array of adaptive equipment and assistive technology options, each contributing to the empowerment of stroke survivors in their pursuit of greater independence and enhanced safety.

Mobility Aids

1. **Canes:** The stalwart cane, available in various configurations such as standard, quad, and offset, is a trusty companion for those with mild balance or gait issues. Adjustable canes offer not only support but also customization, ensuring a comfortable fit tailored to individual needs.

2. **Walkers:** Walkers, spanning standard, two-wheeled, and four-wheeled variations, bestow enhanced stability and weight-bearing support. Some models even incorporate built-in seats, providing users the convenience of resting when required.

3. **Wheelchairs:** Wheelchairs emerge as vital mobility solutions for individuals grappling with profound mobility challenges. Manual wheelchairs, operated by users or caregivers, coexist with power wheelchairs, electrically driven and profoundly liberating.

4. **Mobility Scooters:** Navigating longer distances becomes a reality with battery-powered mobility scooters, available in diverse sizes and styles to accommodate unique requirements.

5. **Transfer Aids:** Facilitating seamless transitions between surfaces, transfer boards, swivel cushions, and transfer belts

redefine safety and ease during transfers, whether from a wheelchair to a bed or from one chair to another.

Adaptive Utensils and Tools

1. **Adaptive Utensils:** These innovative culinary companions, boasting ergonomic designs and easily graspable handles, empower stroke survivors with limited hand dexterity to regain autonomy during mealtimes. The repertoire includes adaptive forks, spoons, and knives, each designed with precision.

2. **Plate Guards and Non-Slip Mats:** Mealtimes are further enhanced with plate guards, which attach to plates to curtail food spillage, and non-slip mats, offering steadfast stability.

3. **Reachers and Grabbers:** Reachers and grabbers extend an invaluable helping hand to individuals with limited reach, enabling them to retrieve items from the floor or reach high shelves with unparalleled ease.

4. **Electric Can Openers:** The chore of opening cans is transformed into a breeze with electric can openers, sparing users the rigors of manual twisting and turning.

Communication Devices

1. **Augmentative and Alternative Communication (AAC) Devices:** A boon for those grappling with speech impediments, AAC devices empower effective expression. They encompass

fundamental communication boards adorned with images to sophisticated speech-generating devices flaunting customizable vocabularies.

2. **Voice Recognition Software:** Voice recognition software, exemplified by Dragon NaturallySpeaking, fosters computer control and text dictation through seamless voice commands.

3. **Tablet Apps:** The digital realm boasts an arsenal of tablet apps catering to diverse communication needs. From text-to-speech applications to symbol-based communication tools, stroke survivors are presented with a multifaceted toolbox.

4. **Electronic Organizers:** Electronic organizers and digital notepads prove indispensable for managing appointments, tasks, and notes. They deftly compensate for memory-related challenges, ensuring no important detail goes unnoticed.

Safety Devices

1. **Home Monitoring Systems:** A vigilant sentry for the home, monitoring systems incorporate video cameras, motion sensors, and alarms, infusing an added layer of safety and security.

2. **Medical Alert Systems:** Wearable medical alert devices, adorned with a call button, offer the assurance of prompt assistance during emergencies, alleviating concerns and bolstering peace of mind.

3. **Fall Detection Devices:** These astute devices automatically dispatch alerts to caregivers or emergency services upon detecting a fall, even in situations where users cannot manually trigger a distress signal.

4. **Adaptive Lighting:** Adaptive lighting systems adjust brightness and color to enhance visibility and safety within the home environment, a crucial asset for stroke survivors.

Cognitive Support Tools

1. **Memory Aids:** Electronic reminders, voice memos, and note-taking apps coalesce to serve as memory aids, offering robust support in memory recall and organization. Vital information, appointments, and tasks are effortlessly retained.

2. **Cognitive Rehabilitation Software:** Cognitive rehabilitation software is a treasure trove of exercises and games meticulously designed to hone memory, attention, and problem-solving skills. It serves as a cornerstone in the journey to cognitive recovery.

3. **Electronic Pill Dispensers:** Seamlessly integrating medication management into daily life, electronic pill dispensers dispense doses at predetermined intervals and accompany this with audible reminders, obviating concerns about missed medications.

Environmental Control Devices

1. **Smart Home Technology:** The era of smart homes unfolds, enabling users to exercise command over lighting, thermostats, door locks, and appliances through the sheer power of voice commands or mobile apps. Independence and convenience merge seamlessly.

2. **Environmental Control Units (ECUs):** ECUs usher in a new era of control for individuals with limited mobility. These devices, operational through switches, voice commands, or head-controlled interfaces, extend authority over various appliances and devices.

3. **Voice-Activated Assistants:** The likes of Amazon Alexa and Google Home usher in an era of unparalleled convenience. Setting reminders, accessing weather updates, and acquiring answers to queries are streamlined, accentuating autonomy.

Computer Accessibility Tools

1. **Ergonomic Keyboards and Mice:** Ergonomically designed keyboards and mice redefine the contours of comfort during computer use. They are especially beneficial for stroke survivors contending with hand and wrist challenges.

2. **Screen Readers and Magnifiers:** Screen readers transmute on-screen text into spoken words, rendering computers accessible

to those with visual impairments. Screen magnifiers step in to amplify on-screen content, ensuring enhanced visibility.

3. **Eye-Tracking Technology:** A technological marvel, eye-tracking technology simplifies computer and device control via eye movements, delivering respite to individuals with limited manual dexterity.

4. **Adaptive Software:** Adaptive software runs the gamut from screen magnification tools to text-to-speech applications. Each one ensures that digital content is effortlessly accessible.

5. **Switch Access Devices:** Pioneering switch access devices open up a world of possibilities for individuals with constrained motor function. These devices facilitate computer and device control through switches activated by various body movements.

The selection of adaptive equipment and assistive technology is a profoundly individualized endeavor, one that meticulously considers individual needs, preferences, and capabilities. The guidance of occupational therapists and rehabilitation specialists proves invaluable in this journey. By embracing these ingenious tools, stroke survivors not only regain control over their lives but also affirm their independence and self-assurance in daily living. Ultimately, these devices enrich overall well-being and elevate the quality of life, propelling stroke survivors towards a future that brims with possibilities.

Diet and Nutrition for Stroke Recovery

The journey of stroke recovery is marked by a multitude of challenges, but few are as crucial as the role of diet and nutrition. Your dietary choices not only impact your physical recovery but also play a pivotal role in preventing secondary strokes and promoting overall well-being. In this comprehensive exploration, we'll delve into the intricate world of diet and nutrition, providing a wealth of information to empower you in making informed decisions that will optimize your stroke recovery journey.

Heart-Healthy Dietary Recommendations

A heart-healthy diet is the linchpin of stroke recovery and prevention. Let's dive into a detailed breakdown of key dietary recommendations:

1. **Fruits and Vegetables:** These colorful powerhouses are packed with essential vitamins, minerals, antioxidants, and dietary fiber. They fortify your immune system, aid digestion, and support overall health. Aim to fill at least half your plate with these nutrient-rich foods. Experiment with a variety of fruits and vegetables to maximize the range of benefits they offer.

2. **Whole Grains:** Whole grains like brown rice, whole wheat bread, quinoa, and oatmeal are rich sources of fiber and complex carbohydrates. They provide sustained energy, regulate blood

sugar levels, and promote cardiovascular health. Opt for whole grains over refined versions to harness their full nutritional potential.

3. **Healthy Fats:** Prioritize unsaturated fats, such as those found in olive oil, avocados, nuts, and fatty fish like salmon, mackerel, and trout. These fats actively work to lower bad cholesterol levels and reduce the risk of heart disease. Incorporate them into your cooking and meal preparation to reap their benefits.

4. **Lean Proteins:** Lean protein sources include skinless poultry, fish, beans, legumes, tofu, and low-fat dairy products. Protein is essential for tissue repair and muscle strength, both crucial components of stroke recovery. Diversify your protein choices to ensure a well-rounded diet.

5. **Limit Sodium:** Excessive sodium intake can elevate blood pressure, increasing the risk of recurrent strokes. Be vigilant about sodium content in foods by reading labels and selecting low-sodium options. Reducing the use of table salt is also advisable.

6. **Control Sugar:** Added sugars found in sugary drinks, sweets, and processed snacks can contribute to weight gain and other health issues. Minimize your consumption of these items, and instead, focus on natural sugars derived from fruits. Pay

attention to concealed sugars in foods that may appear to be nutritious.

7. **Moderate Alcohol:** If you consume alcohol, do so in moderation. For most individuals, moderation translates to up to one drink per day for women and up to two drinks per day for men. Excessive alcohol consumption can lead to high blood pressure and an increased risk of stroke. Remember that abstaining from alcohol is also a valid choice, particularly if you have concerns about its impact on your health.

Portion Control

Portion control is a cornerstone of maintaining a balanced diet. It ensures that you're meeting your nutritional needs without overindulging. Here are practical tips to master portion control:

- Utilize smaller plates and utensils: Smaller tableware naturally limits portion sizes, helping you avoid overeating.
- Mindful eating: Pay attention to your body's hunger and fullness cues. Consuming your meal at a leisurely pace and relishing every mouthful can assist you in identifying when you're content, thus avoiding overindulgence.
- Pre-portion snacks: Divide snacks into appropriate servings beforehand to avoid mindless eating straight from the package.
- Restaurant awareness: Restaurants often serve larger portions than necessary. Consider sharing a meal with a dining

companion or requesting a to-go box to enjoy the remainder later.

Hydration

Proper hydration is a foundational pillar of health and recovery, yet it's frequently underestimated. Water plays a multifaceted role in your body, from aiding digestion and circulation to regulating body temperature. It's crucial to ensure you drink enough water throughout the day. If you face challenges with swallowing or managing fluid intake, consult a speech therapist or healthcare provider for guidance tailored to your specific needs.

Sample Meal Plans

While every individual's dietary needs are unique, here are three sample meal plans adhering to heart-healthy guidelines:

Sample Meal Plan 1

Breakfast:

- Greek yogurt with fresh berries and a sprinkle of almonds.

- Whole grain toast with avocado.

Lunch:

- Salad featuring grilled chicken, a blend of fresh greens, cherry tomatoes, cucumber, and balsamic vinaigrette.

- A serving of quinoa.

Snack:

- Carrot and cucumber sticks with hummus.

Dinner:

- Baked salmon with lemon and dill.

- Steamed broccoli and brown rice.

Snack (if needed):

- A small apple or a handful of grapes.

Sample Meal Plan 2

Breakfast:

- Oatmeal topped with sliced banana and walnuts.

- Low-fat milk or dairy-free alternative.

Lunch:

- Lentil soup.

- Whole grain crackers with sliced cheese and baby carrots.

Snack:

- A piece of fruit (e.g., an orange or a pear).

Dinner:

- Grilled tofu or skinless chicken breast.

- Roasted sweet potatoes and mixed vegetables.

Snack (if needed):

- A small serving of low-fat yogurt.

Sample Meal Plan 3

Breakfast:

- Scrambled eggs with spinach and tomatoes.

- Whole grain toast with a thin layer of peanut butter.

Lunch:

- Quinoa and black bean salad with a lime-cilantro dressing.

- Sliced cucumbers and red bell peppers.

Snack:

- A handful of mixed nuts and dried fruits.

Dinner:

- Baked cod with a lemon-herb marinade.

- Steamed asparagus and quinoa.

Snack (if needed):

- A small serving of cottage cheese with fresh pineapple.

Consulting with Healthcare Professionals

Before embarking on significant dietary changes, especially if you have specific medical conditions, dietary restrictions, or are on medication, it's essential to consult with a healthcare professional or a registered dietitian. These experts can provide personalized guidance tailored to your unique needs, monitor your progress, and adjust your nutrition plan as necessary. Additionally, they can attend to any inquiries or issues you might have about your dietary choices.

In conclusion, diet and nutrition are fundamental pillars of stroke recovery and secondary stroke prevention. By embracing a heart-healthy diet, mastering portion control, staying adequately hydrated, and seeking professional guidance, you empower yourself to embark on a journey of wellness and vitality. Your dietary choices are not merely sustenance but a powerful tool for reclaiming your health and well-being. Every meal is an opportunity to invest in your future and savor the benefits of mindful nutrition, guiding you toward a vibrant life after stroke.

Preventing Secondary Strokes

The journey of stroke recovery is a profound one, marked by resilience, adaptation, and an unwavering commitment to regaining control of one's life. While the process of recovery is often met with its share of challenges, it also presents opportunities for individuals to take proactive steps toward preventing secondary strokes. In this comprehensive guide, we delve into the critical strategies and lifestyle adjustments that can serve as protective measures against the recurrence of stroke, allowing you to chart a course toward a healthier, stroke-free future.

Medication Adherence

One of the cornerstones of stroke prevention is adherence to prescribed medications. If you've been prescribed medications to manage conditions such as high blood pressure, high cholesterol, diabetes, or atrial fibrillation, it's crucial to follow your healthcare provider's instructions meticulously. These medications work to control risk factors associated with stroke and play an integral role in preventing secondary strokes.

- **Stay Organized:** Create a medication schedule or use pill organizers to ensure you take your medications as prescribed.
- **Set Reminders:** Use alarms or smartphone apps to remind you of medication times.
- **Communicate:** If you experience side effects or have concerns about your medications, don't hesitate to discuss them with your healthcare provider. They can explore alternative options or adjust your treatment plan as needed.

Blood Pressure Management

High blood pressure (hypertension) is a significant risk factor for stroke. Managing your blood pressure within a healthy range is paramount in preventing both primary and secondary strokes.

- **Monitor Regularly:** Keep track of your blood pressure at home if recommended by your healthcare provider.
- **Lifestyle Modifications:** Implement lifestyle changes, such as a heart-healthy diet, regular exercise, stress reduction techniques, and limiting alcohol intake, to help manage your blood pressure.
- **Medications:** If prescribed antihypertensive medications, take them consistently and as directed.

Smoking Cessation

Tobacco use is a well-established risk factor for stroke. Smoking not only damages blood vessels but also increases the likelihood of clot formation. Quitting smoking is one of the most impactful steps you can take to reduce your risk of both primary and secondary strokes.

- **Seek Support:** Consider enlisting the help of a smoking cessation program or support group.
- **Nicotine Replacement Therapy:** Nicotine replacement products, such as nicotine gum or patches, can aid in managing withdrawal symptoms.

- **Prescription Medications:** Consult with a healthcare provider about prescription medications that can assist in quitting.

Regular Follow-Up with Healthcare Providers

Consistent follow-up with your healthcare providers is essential for ongoing stroke prevention and management. These visits allow your medical team to monitor your progress, adjust treatment plans as needed, and address any emerging health concerns.

- **Schedule Routine Check-ups:** Attend regular appointments with your primary care physician, neurologist, and any other specialists involved in your care.
- **Communication:** Open and honest communication with your healthcare team is crucial. Share any changes in your health status, symptoms, or concerns during these visits.
- **Compliance:** Follow recommended guidelines for check-ups, screenings, and laboratory tests.

Lifestyle Modifications

In addition to medication adherence and medical management, certain lifestyle modifications can further fortify your defense against secondary strokes:

- **Dietary Choices:** Maintain a heart-healthy diet rich in fruits, vegetables, whole grains, lean proteins, and healthy fats. Minimize sodium and sugar intake.

- **Physical Activity:** Engage in regular physical activity, as approved by your healthcare provider. Exercise helps control risk factors, such as high blood pressure and obesity.

- **Stress Reduction:** Implement stress reduction techniques, such as mindfulness meditation, yoga, or deep breathing exercises, to mitigate stress, which can elevate blood pressure.

- **Moderate Alcohol Consumption:** If you consume alcohol, do so in moderation, following recommended guidelines.

- **Weight Management:** Maintain a healthy weight through a combination of balanced nutrition and physical activity.

Stroke Education and Awareness:

Knowledge is a potent tool in stroke prevention. Educate yourself about the warning signs of stroke and the importance of seeking immediate medical attention if you or someone you know experiences it. Remember the FAST acronym:

- **Face:** Look for facial drooping.

- **Arms:** Examine if there's a downward drift of one arm when it's raised.

- **Speech:** Listen for slurred or garbled speech.

- **Time:** Act quickly; time is critical in stroke care.

By being well-informed and proactive, you empower yourself to recognize and respond to stroke symptoms promptly.

Support Networks

Engage with support networks, such as stroke survivor groups, to connect with individuals who have shared experiences. These communities offer emotional support, valuable insights, and a sense of belonging, enhancing your overall well-being and stroke prevention efforts.

Preventing secondary strokes is a steadfast commitment to your health and future. By adhering to medication regimens, managing blood pressure, quitting smoking, attending regular healthcare appointments, embracing a heart-healthy lifestyle, staying informed, and seeking support, you are taking proactive steps towards a life free from the shadow of stroke. Stroke prevention is a journey that you embark on daily, and your choices today shape your path to a healthier, stroke-resistant tomorrow. With determination, knowledge, and the support of your healthcare team, you can take charge of your destiny and live a vibrant, stroke-free life.

CONCLUSION

As we conclude this journey through the pages of "Stroke Recovery Roadmap," it's crucial to recognize that stroke recovery is not just about the destination; it's about the path you take and the transformative power of each step along the way. Throughout this guide, we've explored the challenges, triumphs, and invaluable guidance needed to navigate the intricate terrain of stroke recovery. Now, as you stand at the intersection of your past and your future, let us reflect on the vital aspects that will continue to shape your journey moving forward.

Recovery, much like life itself, is filled with both small victories and larger milestones. As you travel the road to recovery, take the time to celebrate these accomplishments, no matter how modest they may seem. Whether it's regaining strength in a weakened limb, mastering a new skill, or simply finding joy in everyday moments, these small wins are the building blocks of progress and the sources of inspiration that will propel you forward.

Your support network—comprising family, friends, healthcare professionals, and fellow survivors—has played an essential role in your journey thus far. Nurture and sustain these connections as you move forward. Lean on your loved ones for encouragement, share your experiences and insights with others on a similar path, and continue collaborating with your healthcare team. Remember, you are not alone in this journey, and the bonds you've forged can provide immeasurable strength.

Knowledge is empowerment. As you look toward the future, commit to staying informed about the latest advancements in stroke care, rehabilitation techniques, and preventive measures. Advocate for your health by actively participating in your care decisions, asking questions, and seeking second opinions when necessary. You are your best advocate, and your journey to optimal health relies on your active engagement in your well-being.

In these concluding moments, remember that your journey does not conclude with this book. It continues with every sunrise, every new challenge, and every opportunity to create a life that celebrates your resilience. You've demonstrated remarkable courage, determination, and adaptability—qualities that will continue to serve you well in the days and years ahead. The road to recovery is marked by both triumphs and tribulations, but it is a path illuminated by the indomitable spirit within you.

Stroke recovery is not just about regaining what was lost; it's about discovering the extraordinary potential within you to create a life that is even more fulfilling and vibrant than before. Embrace the unknown with unwavering hope, for the future is brimming with possibilities waiting to be explored. You are the author of your own story, and your resilience is your pen. Write a narrative filled with courage, optimism, and unwavering determination.

In closing, let us remember that stroke recovery is not a solitary endeavor but a collective journey shared by countless individuals who have faced and conquered adversity. As you continue along your unique path, remember that you are part of a community that celebrates strength, perseverance, and the unwavering human spirit. Each chapter of this book has been a guide, a source of knowledge, and a testament to the remarkable journey of stroke recovery. But your story, your journey, and your life beyond stroke are the true epilogue to this book. May your future be filled with renewed vitality, profound joy, and the boundless possibilities that await.

With profound admiration for your resilience and heartfelt best wishes for your continued journey,

Brenda Alderson.

Dear Reader,

I want to extend my heartfelt gratitude for choosing "Stroke Recovery Roadmap" as your companion on your journey to recovery. Your commitment to understanding stroke recovery and your dedication to improving your well-being are truly commendable.

I hope the information and insights shared in this book have proven valuable, offering guidance and support as you progress along your path to recovery. Your pursuit of knowledge and your unwavering determination to regain your health are truly inspiring.

I kindly ask for your support in leaving an honest review of this book. Your feedback will not only help me better understand your experience but also assist other readers who are seeking guidance in their stroke recovery. Your review has the power to make a meaningful difference in their lives.

I want to express my gratitude once more for your presence on this journey. I wish you continued progress, strength, and resilience as you navigate the road to recovery.

With warm regards,

Brenda Alderson.